Bariatric Meal Prep Cookbook

365 Days of Healthy & Easy Recipes and Meal Plans to Enjoy Favorite Foods & Keep the Weight Off

Nigla Muthe

Table of Contents

Introduction

Eating healthy to lose weight doesn't have to mean spending tons of money or hours in the kitchen every day. Bariatric Meal Prep Cookbook teaches you how to prepare healthy meals in efficient batches so you can enjoy them all week long. With these meal plans and recipes, you'll always have a fast, nourishing meal to reach for—helping you feel great and lose weight sustainably, week after week.

Learn the basics of meal planning and quick, consistent food preparation. Each plan includes shopping lists, recipes, and step-by-step instructions for meal prep. Most of the batch-friendly recipes all include nutritional information, so you can easily swap them into your meal plans. Stay on track to your weight loss goals with the perfectly portioned meal prep plans in this Bariatric Meal Prep Cookbook.

Chapter 1: Overview of Bariatric Diet

What is Bariatric Diet?

A bariatric surgery, such as a gastric bypass, is a major procedure that requires a strict diet, especially during recovery.

It is meant to help you lose the extra weight by making adjustments to your digestive system.

A bariatric diet is intended to aid in the healing process and provide support in establishing new habits that are suitable for a healthier lifestyle.

General Guidelines for Following the Bariatric Diet

A bariatric procedure may decrease the size of your stomach (to about the size of a walnut), reduce your ability to absorb nutrients, inhibit the hormone ghrelin (the hunger hormone), and shorten the pathway of food through the intestines.

The body will need ample time to heal and adjust to these changes. A bariatric diet follows a progression from liquids, pureed, soft foods, and regular foods.

Below are some of the guidelines that your doctor might recommend while on a bariatric diet.

- Drink enough water within the day.
- Drink your liquids slowly. Avoid using straws or drinking carbonated drinks.
- Drink a cup of water or fluid only between meals and not during. Ideally, drink only 30 minutes after your meal.
- Follow the proposed portion size for each stage and monitor your daily intake.
- Eat food slowly and chew thoroughly.
- Eat balanced meals that are within your suggested daily calorie intake.
- Take the recommended multivitamins or supplements. Typically, you will be asked to take calcium, vitamin D, vitamin b12, iron, and folic acid supplements depending on your needs.

Foods to Eat

Immediately following the surgery, you will be required by your doctor to undergo a clear liquid diet for the first few days.

Below are examples of foods that you should eat:

- Fat-free, protein-rich foods like soft scrambled eggs, lean poultry, lean ground meat, lean fish, and seafood
- Vegetables that are fully cooked and without their skin
- Canned fruits
- Beans and peas
- Non-fat yogurt, cottage cheese, and other milk derivatives, as long as you can tolerate them.

After weeks of recovery, you can start to gradually go back to your normal diet. But of course, it's imperative that you make healthier choices.

Your diet must now consist of:

- Plenty fruits and vegetables
- Lean meat and poultry
- Whole grains
- Healthy fats
- Seafood
- Nuts and seeds (crushed or softened)

Foods to Avoid

Aside from knowing which foods to eat, it is equally important to know and understand which foods you need to avoid.

Here are some foods you should steer clear of:

- Foods and beverages that have a high amount of sugars, calories, or fats
- Foods that are rich in carbohydrates like white rice, bread, and pasta
- Alcohol and caffeine
- Raw or partially cooked vegetables (abstain eating cabbage, corn, celery, and other similar fibrous vegetables)
- Fresh fruits with skins and seeds
- Red meat and tough meats
- Spicy foods or those with lots of seasonings
- Dry foods like nuts, granola, and seeds
- Fried food

Chapter 2: 4-Week Prep Plans to Start Your Journey

Week 1

Sunday

Breakfast: Cottage cheese pancake

Lunch: Pureed carrot

Dinner: Zucchini soup with rosemary

Monday

Breakfast: Baked eggs with broccoli

Lunch: Pumpkin puree

Dinner: Chicken tikka masala

Tuesday

Breakfast: Breakfast popsicle

Lunch: Cream of asparagus soup

Dinner: Tofu & quinoa bowl

Wednesday

Breakfast: Pumpkin oatmeal

Lunch: Roasted sweet potato puree

Dinner: Crispy chicken

Thursday

Breakfast: Breakfast strawberry wrap

Lunch: Ginger beef stir fry

Dinner: Mushroom soup

Friday

Breakfast: Baked eggs with broccoli

Lunch: Mashed parsnips

Dinner: Creamy chicken

Saturday

Breakfast: Baked spinach & cottage cheese

Lunch: Celery root puree

Dinner: Cajun chicken

Week 2

Sunday

Breakfast: Breakfast enchilada

Lunch: Baked chicken & vegetables

Dinner: Hummus

Monday

Breakfast: Pumpkin oatmeal

Lunch: Creamy acorn squash soup

Dinner: Tofu & quinoa bowl

Tuesday

Breakfast: Breakfast sandwich

Lunch: Roasted sweet potato puree

Dinner: Chicken tikka masala

Wednesday

Breakfast: Broccoli & tofu scramble

Lunch: Kale soup with white beans

Dinner: Asian-style pork tenderloin

Thursday

Breakfast: Cottage cheese pancake

Lunch: Crispy tuna patties

Dinner: Tomato soup

Week 3

Sunday

Breakfast: Breakfast enchilada

Lunch: Tofu & quinoa bowl

Dinner: Fried trout

Monday

Breakfast: Baked spinach & cottage cheese

Lunch: Butternut squash & coconut milk soup

Dinner: Pork & black bean stew

Tuesday

Breakfast: Cottage cheese pancake

Lunch: Barbecue salmon

Dinner: Chicken & broccoli soup

Wednesday

Breakfast: Breakfast sandwich

Friday

Breakfast: Egg muffin

Lunch: Creamy chicken

Dinner: Ginger beef stir fry

Saturday

Breakfast: Breakfast popsicle

Lunch: Chicken casserole

Dinner: Mushroom soup

Lunch: Chicken casserole

Dinner: Tomato soup

Thursday

Breakfast: Breakfast popsicle

Lunch: Broccoli puree

Dinner: Greek chicken

Friday

Breakfast: Broccoli & tofu scramble

Lunch: Crispy tuna patties

Dinner: Potato soup

Saturday

Breakfast: Egg muffin

Lunch: Chicken & broccoli soup

Dinner: Fried trout

Week 4

Sunday

Breakfast: Breakfast strawberry wrap

Lunch: Barbecue salmon

Dinner: Butternut squash & coconut milk soup

Monday

Breakfast: Breakfast sandwich

Lunch: Greek chicken

Dinner: Potato soup

Tuesday

Breakfast: Breakfast enchilada

Lunch: Sweet & sour pork

Dinner: Creamy cauliflower puree

Wednesday

Breakfast: Baked eggs with broccoli

Lunch: Chicken casserole

Dinner: Pureed carrot

Thursday

Breakfast: Baked spinach & cottage cheese

Lunch: Broccoli puree

Dinner: Fried trout

Friday

Breakfast: Egg muffin

Lunch: Crispy tuna patties

Dinner: Carrot & parsnip puree

Saturday

Breakfast: Pumpkin oatmeal

Lunch: Creamy cauliflower puree

Dinner: Pork & black bean stew

Chapter 3: Breakfast

Cottage Cheese Pancake

Preparation Time: 5 minutes
Cooking Time: 5 minutes
Servings: 4

Ingredients:

- ½ tsp baking soda
- ⅓ cup all-purpose flour
- 1 cup low-fat cottage cheese
- 3 eggs, beaten
- ½ tablespoon oil

Method:

1. Mix all ingredients except oil in a bowl.
2. Add oil to the pan over medium heat.
3. Store batter in a food container.
4. Refrigerate until ready to cook.
5. When ready to cook, pour batter into the pan.
6. Flip once bubbles appear.
7. Cook for 2 to 3 minutes or until firm.

Nutritional Content:

- Calories: 152
- Fat: 7 g
- Cholesterol: 2 mg
- Carbohydrate: 10 g
- Sodium: 385 mg
- Sugar: 2 g
- Protein: 13 g

Breakfast Enchilada

Preparation Time: 5 minutes
Cooking Time: 3 minutes
Servings: 1

Ingredients:

- 1 egg white, beaten
- 1 egg, beaten
- Cooking spray
- Salt and pepper to taste
- 1 oz. tofu, sliced into cubes and cooked
- 2 tablespoons salsa
- 1 tablespoon low-fat Mexican cheese, shredded

Method:

1. Mix egg white and egg in a bowl.
2. Spray a pan with oil.
3. Place the pan over medium heat.
4. Add the eggs and cook for 1 to 2 minutes without stirring.
5. Season with salt and pepper.
6. Flip and cook for another 1 minute.
7. Transfer to a plate.
8. Cook eggs on the other side about two minutes or until completely cooked and transfer to a plate.
9. Top the egg with tofu and cheese.
10. Roll it up.
11. Store in a food container.
12. Refrigerate for up to 1 day.
13. Reheat when ready to serve.
14. Serve with salsa.

Nutritional Content:

- Calories: 171
- Fat: 8 g
- Cholesterol: 0 mg
- Carbohydrate: 3 g
- Protein: 23 g
- Sodium: 432 mg
- Sugar: 3 g

Baked Eggs with Broccoli

Preparation Time: 15 minutes
Cooking Time: 1 hour and 30 minutes
Servings: 8

Ingredients:

- 1 teaspoon olive oil
- 6 eggs, beaten
- ½ cup mushrooms, sliced
- 10 oz. broccoli florets, chopped
- Pinch paprika
- Salt and pepper to taste

Method:

1. Preheat your oven to 350 degrees F.
2. Mix all ingredients in a bowl.
3. Add mixture to a baking pan.
4. Bake in the oven for 1 hour and 30 minutes.
5. Store in food container and refrigerate.
6. Reheat before serving.

Nutritional Content:

- Calories: 115
- Fat: 5 g
- Cholesterol: 75 mg
- Carbohydrate: 5 g
- Sodium: 419 mg
- Sugar: 2 g
- Protein: 12 g

Broccoli & Tofu Scramble

Preparation Time: 10 minutes
Cooking Time: 10 minutes
Servings: 6

Ingredients:

- 1 tablespoon oil
- 1 onion, chopped
- ¼ lb. mushrooms, chopped
- ½ lb. broccoli, chopped
- 1½ lb. tofu, sliced into cubes
- 3 eggs, beaten

Method:

1. Preheat your oven to 350 degrees F.
2. Add oil to a pan over medium heat.
3. Cook onion and mushrooms for 1 minute.
4. Push to one side.
5. Add tofu and broccoli.
6. Cook until tofu cubes are golden.
7. Add mixture to a bowl with the eggs.
8. Put the egg mixture back to the pan.
9. Cook until eggs are set.
10. Store in food container and refrigerate.

Nutritional Content:

- Calories: 190
- Fat: 8g
- Cholesterol: 0 mg
- Sodium: 350 mg
- Carbohydrates: 18g
- Dietary fiber: 4g
- Sugar: 3g
- Protein: 13g

Breakfast Sandwich

Preparation Time: 5 minutes
Cooking Time: 0 minute
Servings: 3

Ingredients:

- 1 apple, chopped
- 6 oz. canned tuna flakes in water, drained
- 1 teaspoon mustard
- ¼ cup low-fat vanilla yogurt
- 6 slices whole wheat bread
- 3 lettuces leaves

Method:

1. Mix apple, tuna flakes, mustard and yogurt in a bowl.
2. Spread mixture on top of the 3 bread slices.
3. Add lettuce and top with the other bread slice.
4. Store in food container.
5. Refrigerate for up to 1 day.

Nutritional Content:

- Calories: 250
- Fat: 2.5 g
- Cholesterol: 28 mg
- Sodium: 330 mg
- Carbohydrates: 30 g
- Sugar: 5.25 g
- Dietary Fiber: 5 g
- Protein: 23 g

Breakfast Strawberry Wrap

Preparation Time: 5 minutes
Cooking Time: 0 minute
Servings: 1

Ingredients:

- 1 whole wheat tortilla
- 1 tablespoon low-sugar strawberry jam
- 3 tablespoons ricotta cheese
- ¼ cup strawberries, sliced

Method:

1. Spread the tortilla with strawberry jam and ricotta cheese.
2. Top with the strawberry slices.
3. Roll up.
4. Store in food container and refrigerate.

Nutritional Content:

- Calories: 233
- Fat: 9 g
- Cholesterol: 24 mg
- Carbohydrate: 30 g
- Sodium: 229 mg
- Sugar: 8 g
- Protein: 8 g

Breakfast Popsicle

Preparation Time: 5 hours and 5 minutes
Cooking Time: 0 minute
Servings: 6

Ingredients:

- 1 cup plain Greek yogurt (non-fat)
- ½ cup almond milk
- ½ cup oats
- 1 cup mixed berries

Method:

1. Combine all ingredients.
2. Pour mixture into popsicle molds.
3. Freeze for 5 hours.
4. Serve when ready to eat.

Nutritional Content:

- Calories: 75
- Fat: 0.6 g
- Cholesterol: 3 mg
- Sodium: 36 mg
- Carbohydrates: 11 g
- Dietary Fiber: 1.5 g
- Sugar: 4 g
- Protein: 5 g

Pumpkin Oatmeal

Preparation Time: 5 minutes
Cooking Time: 3 minutes
Servings: 1

Ingredients:

- ¼ cup rolled oats
- ⅛ teaspoon cinnamon
- ½ cup pumpkin puree
- Pinch ground ginger
- Pinch ground cloves
- ½ cup salt-free cottage cheese
- 1 teaspoon Truvia baking blend

Method:

1. Add all ingredients except cheese to a microwave-safe dish or bowl.
2. Mix well.
3. Microwave on high setting for 80 to 90 seconds.
4. Add cottage cheese. Microwave on high for 1 minute
5. Store in a glass jar with lid and refrigerate for up to 1 day.

Nutritional Content:

- Calories: 205
- Fat: 3 g
- Cholesterol: 3 mg
- Sodium: 312 mg
- Carbohydrates: 34 g
- Dietary Fiber: 7 g
- Sugar: 9 g
- Protein: 14 g

Egg Muffin

Preparation Time: 10 minutes
Cooking Time: 20 minutes
Servings: 12

Ingredients:

- Cooking spray
- 12 turkey bacon slices, cooked and sliced
- 6 eggs, beaten
- ½ cup almond milk
- ¾ cup low-fat Swiss cheese
- ¼ teaspoon Italian seasoning
- Salt and pepper to taste

Method:

1. Spray muffin pan with oil.
2. Preheat your oven to 350 degrees F.
3. Add bacon to the muffin cups.
4. In a bowl, mix the remaining ingredients.
5. Pour mixture into the muffin cups.
6. Bake in the oven for 20 minutes.
7. Transfer egg muffins to food container.
8. Refrigerate for up to 1 day.
9. Reheat before serving.

Nutritional Content:

- Calories: 98
- Fat: 7g
- Cholesterol: 7 mg
- Carbohydrates: 1g
- Fiber: 0g
- Sugar: 1g
- Protein: 8g

Baked Spinach & Cottage Cheese

Preparation Time: 10 minutes
Cooking Time: 30 minutes
Servings: 8

Ingredients:

- 2 cups non-fat cottage cheese
- 2 eggs, beaten
- 10 oz. spinach

Method:

1. Preheat oven to 350 degrees F.
2. Combine cheese, eggs and spinach in a bowl.
3. Pour into a baking pan.
4. Bake for 30 minutes.
5. Store in food container and refrigerate.

Nutritional Content:

- Calories: 78
- Fat: 3 g
- Cholesterol: 0 mg
- Carbohydrates: 3 g
- Fiber: 1 g
- Sugars: 2 g
- Protein: 11 g

Chapter 4: Soup

Tomato Soup

Preparation Time: 10 minutes
Cooking Time: 30 minutes
Servings: 4

Ingredients:

- 1 teaspoon olive oil
- 1 teaspoon garlic, minced
- 14 oz. tomatoes, chopped
- 28 oz. canned tomatoes
- 1 teaspoon Italian seasoning
- ¼ cup Parmesan cheese
- Salt and pepper to taste

Method:

1. Add oil to a pot over medium heat.
2. Add garlic and cook for 30 seconds, stirring often.
3. Add the rest of the ingredients.
4. Simmer for 20 to 25 minutes.
5. Turn off heat.
6. Let cool.
7. Transfer to a food processor.
8. Blend until smooth.
9. Transfer to food container.
10. Freeze until ready to serve.
11. Reheat before serving.

Nutritional Content:

- Calories: 157
- Fat: 3.2
- Cholesterol: 2 mg
- Sodium: 10 mg
- Carbohydrates: 3.2 g
- Fiber: 3 g
- Sugar: 5 g
- Protein: 24 g

Chicken & Broccoli Soup

Preparation Time: 20 minutes
Cooking Time: 40 minutes
Servings: 6

Ingredients:

- Cooking spray
- ½ cup onion, chopped
- ½ cup celery, chopped
- 1 cup broccoli florets, chopped
- ½ cup carrot, chopped
- 4 cups reduced-sodium chicken stock
- ½ teaspoon dried basil
- ½ teaspoon dried oregano
- ½ teaspoon dried thyme
- 1 lb. chicken breasts, cooked and shredded
- 12 oz. milk
- 1 tablespoon Worcestershire sauce

Method:

1. Spray your pot with oil.
2. Place pot over medium heat.
3. Add onion, celery, broccoli and carrot to the pot.
4. Cook for 5 minutes.
5. Add stock and dried herbs.
6. Simmer for 15 to 20 minutes.
7. Add milk, chicken and Worcestershire sauce.
8. Cook for 5 minutes.

Nutritional Content:

- Calories: 260
- Fat: 2.5 g
- Cholesterol: 20 mg
- Sodium: 12 mg
- Carbohydrates: 25 g
- Fiber: 6 g
- Sugar: 8.5 g
- Protein: 31 g

Zucchini Soup with Rosemary

Preparation Time: 30 minutes
Cooking Time: 40 minutes
Servings: 8

Ingredients:

- 1 tablespoon vegetable oil
- 2 tablespoons butter
- 1 onion, chopped
- 2 teaspoons fresh rosemary, minced
- 2 cloves garlic, sliced
- 1 potato, sliced
- 4 cups vegetable broth
- 3 zucchinis, sliced
- Green onions, chopped

Method:

1. Add oil and butter to a pan over medium high heat.
2. Cook onion for 5 minutes.
3. Stir in rosemary and garlic.
4. Cook for 2 minutes.
5. Add potato and broth.
6. Bring to a boil and simmer for 10 minutes.
7. Stir in zucchini and simmer for 15 minutes.
8. Turn off heat.
9. Let cool.
10. Transfer to a food processor.
11. Process until pureed.
12. Reheat.
13. Top with green onions.
14. Transfer to food container.
15. Freeze for up to 1 month.
16. Reheat before serving.

Nutritional Content:

- Calories: 89
- Fat: 2 g
- Cholesterol: 8 mg
- Sodium: 12 mg
- Carbohydrates: 10 g
- Fiber: 2 g
- Sugar: 2.5 g
- Protein: 3 g

Mushroom Soup

Preparation Time: 10 minutes
Cooking Time: 25 minutes
Servings: 2

Ingredients:

- 1 tablespoon coconut oil
- 1 onion, chopped
- 2 cloves garlic, chopped
- 10 ½ oz. mushrooms, sliced
- 1 stalk celery, sliced
- 1 cup vegetable stock
- 1 cup oat milk
- Salt and pepper to taste

Method:

1. Pour oil into a pot over medium heat.
2. Cook onion, garlic, mushrooms and celery for 10 minutes.
3. Stir in the remaining ingredients.
4. Bring to a boil.
5. Simmer for 15 minutes.
6. Turn off heat.
7. Let cool.
8. Transfer to food container.
9. Process until pureed.
10. Store in food container.
11. Freeze for up to 1 month.
12. Reheat before serving.

Nutritional Content:

- Calories: 385
- Fat: 10 g
- Cholesterol: 0 mg
- Sodium: 526 mg
- Carbohydrates: 57 g
- Fiber: 3 g
- Sugar: 6 g
- Protein: 21 g

Creamy Acorn Squash Soup

Preparation Time: 10 minutes
Cooking Time: 40 minutes
Servings: 6

Ingredients:

- 2 tablespoons coconut oil
- 2 onions, sliced
- 3 acorn squash, sliced in half and roasted
- 1 ½ cups vegetable broth
- ¾ cup coconut milk
- 1 tablespoon curry powder

Method:

1. Add coconut oil to a soup pot over medium heat.
2. Cook onion for 1 to 2 minutes.
3. Stir in the squash.
4. Pour in the broth and coconut milk.
5. Add the curry powder.
6. Mix well.
7. Bring to a boil.
8. Simmer for 30 minutes.
9. Turn off heat and let cool.
10. Transfer to a food processor.
11. Process to puree.
12. Store in food containers and freeze for up to 1 month.
13. Reheat when ready to serve.

Nutritional Content:

- Calories: 283
- Fat: 18 g
- Cholesterol: 1 mg
- Sodium: 120 mg
- Carbohydrates: 29 g
- Fiber: 4 g
- Sugar: 2 g
- Protein: 4 g

Butternut Squash & Coconut Milk Soup

Preparation Time: 15 minutes
Cooking Time: 45 minutes
Servings: 6

Ingredients:

- 2 tablespoons olive oil
- 1 white onion, chopped
- 1 ¼ tsp. ginger, crushed
- 3 cloves garlic, crushed
- 1 butternut squash, sliced and roasted
- Salt to taste
- ¼ tsp. cinnamon powder
- 15 oz. coconut milk
- 2 cups vegetable broth

Method:

1. Add olive oil to a pot over medium heat.
2. Cook onion, ginger and garlic for 3 minutes.
3. Stir in butternut squash slices
4. Season with salt and cinnamon powder.
5. Cook for 3 minutes.
6. Pour in milk and broth.
7. Bring to a boil.
8. Simmer for 30 minutes.
9. Turn off heat.
10. Let cool.
11. Transfer to food processor.
12. Pulse until smooth.
13. Transfer to food container.
14. Freeze for up to 1 month.
15. Reheat before serving.

Nutritional Content:

- Calories: 321
- Fat: 3 g

- Cholesterol: 0 mg
- Sodium: 415 mg
- Carbohydrates: 32 g

- Fiber: 5 g
- Sugar: 6 g
- Protein: 4 g

Cream of Asparagus Soup

Preparation Time: 10 minutes
Cooking Time: 20 minutes
Servings: 4

Ingredients:

- 1 tablespoon olive oil
- 1 clove garlic, minced
- 1 onion, sliced
- 1 carrot, chopped
- 1 stalk celery, chopped
- 10 ½ oz. asparagus, chopped
- 2 cups vegetable stock
- 1 cup water
- 1 cup almond milk
- Salt and pepper to taste

Method:

1. Add oil to a pan over medium heat.
2. Cook garlic, onion, carrot and celery for 10 minutes, stirring often.
3. Add asparagus, stock, water and almond milk.
4. Season with salt and pepper.
5. Bring to a boil.
6. Simmer for 10 minutes.
7. Let cool.
8. Transfer to food processor.
9. Pulse until smooth.
10. Freeze for up to 1 month.

Nutritional Content:

- Calories: 203
- Fat: 5 g
- Cholesterol: 0 mg
- Sodium: 262 mg
- Carbohydrates: 29 g
- Fiber: 8 g
- Sugar: 4 g
- Protein: 10 g

Kale Soup with White Beans

Preparation Time: 10 minutes
Cooking Time: 30 minutes
Servings: 4

Ingredients:

- 1 tablespoon avocado oil
- 1 onion, chopped
- 3 stalks celery, chopped
- 3 potatoes, diced
- 3 carrots, chopped
- Salt and pepper to taste
- 4 cloves garlic, minced
- 2 tablespoons Italian seasoning
- 30 oz. white beans, rinsed and drained
- 32 oz. vegetable broth
- 26 oz. canned diced tomatoes
- 1 cup kale, chopped

Method:

1. Pour oil into a pot over medium heat.
2. Cook the onion, celery, carrots and potatoes for 7 to 8 minutes.
3. Season with salt.
4. Add garlic and Italian seasoning.
5. Cook for 1 minute.
6. Add the rest of the ingredients except kale.
7. Bring to a boil.
8. Simmer for 20 minutes.
9. Add kale and cook for 1 minute.
10. Let cool.
11. Store in food containers and freeze for up to 1 month.

Nutritional Content:

- Calories: 309
- Fat: 3 g
- Cholesterol: 0 mg
- Sodium: 126 mg
- Carbohydrates: 57 g
- Fiber: 12 g
- Sugar: 12 g
- Protein: 15 g

Turkey & Corn Soup

Preparation Time: 20 minutes
Cooking Time: 30 minutes
Servings: 6

Ingredients:

- 1 teaspoon olive oil
- 1 onion, diced
- 2 cloves garlic, minced
- 1 red bell pepper, chopped
- 1 stalk celery, diced
- 4 oz. canned diced green chili
- 3 cups reduced-sodium chicken broth
- 1 ¼ cups corn kernels
- 2 cups almond milk
- ¼ cup all-purpose flour
- 2 cups turkey, cooked and shredded
- Green onion, chopped

Method:

1. Add olive oil to a pan over medium heat.
2. Cook onion, garlic, bell pepper and celery for 5 minutes.
3. Stir in green chili.
4. Cook for 1 minute.
5. Add chicken broth.
6. Bring to a boil.
7. Reduce heat and simmer for 10 minutes.
8. Stir in corn and simmer for 5 minutes.
9. Mix milk and flour in a bowl.
10. Add mixture to the soup.
11. Cook for 15 minutes.
12. Add turkey and green onions.
13. Let cool.
14. Transfer to food container.
15. Freeze for up to 1 month.

16. Reheat before serving.

Nutritional Content:

- Calories: 223.3
- Fat: 6.6 g
- Cholesterol: 13 mg
- Sodium: 143 mg
- Carbohydrates: 25 g
- Fiber: 1.6 g
- Sugar: 8.8 g
- Protein: 15.6 g

Potato Soup

Preparation Time: 10 minutes
Cooking Time: 1 hour
Servings: 4

Ingredients:

- Water
- 4 cups potatoes, chopped
- 4 cups vegetable broth
- 1 tablespoon olive oil
- 1 onion, chopped
- Salt and pepper to taste
- Green onions, chopped

Method:

1. Fill a pot with water.
2. Boil potatoes for 20 to 30 minutes.
3. Drain the water.
4. In a pan over medium heat, add the oil and onion.
5. Cook for 3 minutes.
6. Put the potatoes back to the pan along with the broth.
7. Season with salt and pepper.
8. Cover the pot.
9. Cook for 30 minutes.
10. Turn off heat.
11. Let cool.
12. Transfer mixture to a food processor.
13. Puree and store in food containers.
14. Freeze for up to 1 month.
15. Reheat before serving.

Nutritional Content:

- Calories: 12
- Fat: 5 g
- Cholesterol: 0 mg
- Sodium: 21 mg
- Carbohydrates: 24 g
- Fiber: 3 g
- Sugar: 0 g
- Protein: 8 g

Chapter 5: Pureed Food

Pureed Carrot

Preparation Time: 10 minutes
Cooking Time: 30 minutes
Servings: 4

Ingredients:

- 2 lb. carrots, sliced
- Water
- Salt and pepper to taste

Method:

1. Add carrots to a pan over medium heat.
2. Fill pan with water.
3. Bring to a boil.
4. Reduce heat.
5. Simmer for 20 minutes.
6. Drain.
7. Transfer carrots to a blender.
8. Puree until smooth.
9. Season with salt and pepper.

Nutritional Content:

- Calories: 120
- Fat: 4 g
- Cholesterol: 2 mg
- Carbohydrate: 10 g
- Sodium: 200 mg
- Sugar: 2 g
- Protein: 6 g

Mashed Parsnips

Preparation Time: 10 minutes
Cooking Time: 30 minutes
Servings: 8

Ingredients:

- 5 cups nut milk
- 10 parsnips, sliced into cubes
- Salt and pepper to taste
- 1 teaspoon dried thyme

Method:

1. Add milk to a pot over medium heat.
2. Heat for 1 minute.
3. Add parsnips and simmer for 30 minutes.
4. Mash parsnips on a plate.
5. Stir in 1 cup of the warm milk along with the salt, pepper and thyme.
6. Store in food container.
7. Serve within the day.

Nutritional Content:

- Calories: 143.2
- Fat: 10.7 g
- Cholesterol: 30.5 mg
- Sodium: 392.7 mg
- Carbohydrates: 7.1 g
- Fiber: o.1 g
- Sugar: 6.9 g
- Protein: 5 g

Roasted Sweet Potato Puree

Preparation Time: 10 minutes
Cooking Time: 1 hour
Servings: 6

Ingredients:

- Olive oil
- 3 lb. sweet potatoes, sliced
- Pepper to taste

Method:

1. Add sweet potatoes to a baking pan.
2. Drizzle with olive oil.
3. Bake in the oven for 1 hour.
4. Let cool.
5. Transfer to a food processor.
6. Pulse until smooth.
7. Store in food container.
8. Refrigerate for up to 3 days.

Nutritional Content:

- Calories: 238.1
- Fat: 9.4
- Cholesterol: 25 mg
- Sodium: 322 mg
- Carbohydrates: 35.7 g
- Fiber: 5.1 g
- Sugar: 8.5 g
- Protein: 3.8 g

Pumpkin Puree

Preparation Time: 10 minutes
Cooking Time: 1 hour
Servings: 4

Ingredients:

- 1 pumpkin, sliced in half, seeds removed

Method:

1. Preheat your oven to 325 degrees F.
2. Cover the pumpkin with foil.
3. Bake in the oven for 1 hour.
4. Let cool.
5. Scrape the flesh.
6. Add to a food processor.
7. Pulse until smooth.
8. Transfer to food container.
9. Refrigerate for up to 3 days or freeze for up to 1 month.

Nutritional Content:

- Calories: 188
- Fat: 0.7 g
- Cholesterol: 0 mg
- Sodium: 7 mg
- Carbohydrates: 47.2 g
- Fiber: 3.6 g
- Sugar: 9.9 g
- Protein: 7.3 g

Vegetable Puree

Preparation Time: 15 minutes
Cooking Time: 45 minutes
Servings: 8

Ingredients:

- 30 oz. vegetable broth
- 6 oz. mushrooms, sliced
- 1 carrot, sliced
- 1 potato, sliced into cubes
- ½ cup corn kernels
- 1 turnip, sliced into cubes
- ¼ cup cabbage, shredded
- ½ cup green peas
- Pinch Italian seasoning

Method:

1. Boil all the vegetables in the broth for 40 minutes.
2. Drain.
3. Add to a food processor.
4. Pulse until pureed.
5. Sprinkle with Italian seasoning.
6. Transfer to a food container.
7. Refrigerate for up to 3 days.

Nutritional Content:

- Calories: 66.7
- Fat: 0.5
- Cholesterol: 0 mg
- Sodium: 102 mg
- Carbohydrates: 14.1 g
- Fiber: 2.6 g
- Sugar: 4.6 g
- Protein: 2.3 g

Creamy Cauliflower Puree

Preparation Time: 5 minutes
Cooking Time: 0 minute
Servings: 4

Ingredients:

- 4 teaspoons olive oil
- 3 cloves garlic, cooked
- 4 cups cauliflower florets, steamed
- ¼ cup nonfat milk
- ½ teaspoon black pepper
- ½ teaspoon garlic salt

Method:

1. Combine all ingredients to a food processor.
2. Pulse until smooth.
3. Store in an airtight container.
4. Refrigerate for up to 3 days.

Nutritional Content:

- Calories: 113
- Fat: 6 g
- Protein: 5 g
- Carbohydrate: 13 g
- Cholesterol: 3 mg
- Sodium: 383 mg
- Sugar: 6 g

Hummus

Preparation Time: 10 minutes
Cooking Time: 0 minute
Servings: 12

Ingredients:

- 15 oz. chickpeas, rinsed and drained
- 1 clove garlic, crushed
- 3 tablespoons olive oil
- 3 tablespoons lemon juice
- ½ teaspoon salt
- 1 tablespoon tahini

Method:

1. Add all ingredients to a food processor.
2. Process until smooth.
3. Store in an airtight container.
4. Refrigerate for up to 1 week.

Nutritional Content:

- Calories: 72
- Fat: 4.5 g
- Protein: 1.5 g
- Carbohydrate: 7.5 g
- Cholesterol: 0 mg
- Sodium: 149 mg
- Sugar: 0 g

Broccoli Puree

Preparation Time: 10 minutes
Cooking Time: 30 minutes
Servings: 4

Ingredients:

- Water
- 4 cups broccoli florets
- 2 tablespoons vegan butter
- ½ cup heavy cream
- Pinch ground nutmeg

Method:

1. Fill a pot with water.
2. Place it over medium heat.
3. Boil the broccoli for 20 minutes.
4. Drain and rinse.
5. Add to the broccoli to a food processor along with the rest of the ingredients. Pulse until smooth.
6. Store in food container.
7. Refrigerate for up to 3 days.

Nutritional Content:

- Calories: 200
- Fat: 17.4 g
- Cholesterol: 12 mg
- Sodium: 102 mg
- Carbohydrates: 9.9 g
- Fiber: 3.6 g
- Sugar: 2 g
- Protein: 4.5 g

Carrot & Parsnip Puree

Preparation Time: 15 minutes
Cooking Time: 20 minutes
Servings: 4

Ingredients:

- 2 carrots, sliced
- 8 parsnips, sliced into cubes
- Water
- ¼ cup chives, snipped
- 6 tablespoons vegan butter
- Pepper to taste

Method:

1. Add carrots and parsnips to a pot.
2. Cover with water.
3. Boil for 20 minutes. Drain.
4. Mash the vegetables using a potato masher.
5. Stir in remaining ingredients.
6. Transfer to a food container.
7. Refrigerate for up to 3 days.

Nutritional Content:

- Calories: 164.3
- Fat: 0.5 g
- Cholesterol: 45.8 mg
- Sodium: 220.5 mg
- Carbohydrates: 2.7 g
- Fiber: 3 g
- Sugar: 2 g
- Protein: 0.5 g

Celery Root Puree

Preparation Time: 15 minutes
Cooking Time: 15 minutes
Servings: 6

Ingredients:

- 2 tablespoons lemon juice, divided
- 1 celery root, sliced
- Water
- ¼ cup heavy whipping cream
- Pinch cayenne pepper

Method:

1. Add 1 tablespoon lemon juice and celery root to a pot of water.
2. Bring to a boil.
3. Reduce heat.
4. Simmer for 20 minutes.
5. Drain and let cool.
6. Add the mixture to your food processor.
7. Stir in the cream, cayenne pepper and remaining lemon juice.
8. Process until pureed.
9. Store in food container.
10. Refrigerate for up to 3 days.

Nutritional Content:

- Calories: 139.4
- Fat: 2.5 g
- Cholesterol: 28 mg
- Sodium: 232.9 mg
- Carbohydrates: 14.7 g
- Fiber: 3.3 g
- Sugar: 2.2 g
- Protein: 9 g

Chapter 6: Main Dishes

Fried Trout

Preparation Time: 15 minutes
Cooking Time: 10 minutes
Servings: 2

Ingredients:

- 3 tablespoons yellow cornmeal
- ¼ teaspoon ground celery seeds
- 2 tablespoons parsley, chopped
- Pepper to taste
- 2 rainbow trout fillets
- 2 teaspoons olive oil

Method:

1. In a bowl, combine cornmeal, ground celery, parsley and pepper.
2. Coat both sides of the fish with this mixture.
3. Transfer breaded fish to a food container.
4. Freeze for up to 1 month.
5. When ready to cook, add olive oil to a pan over medium heat.
6. Cook in the pan for 3 to 5 minutes per side or until crispy.

Nutritional Content:

- Calories: 240
- Fat: 10g
- Cholesterol: 67mg
- Carbohydrates: 10g
- Sodium: 338mg
- Sugars: 0g
- Protein: 25g

Chicken Tikka Masala

Preparation Time: 20 minutes
Cooking Time: 8 hours
Servings: 10

Ingredients:

- 2 tablespoons olive oil
- 1 onion, diced
- 4 cloves garlic, minced
- 2 tablespoons ginger, minced
- 3 lb. chicken breast fillets, sliced into strips
- 1 ½ cups Greek yogurt
- 29 oz. canned tomato puree
- 1 tablespoon cumin
- 2 tablespoons garam masala
- ¾ teaspoon cinnamon
- ½ tablespoon paprika
- 2 bay leaves
- Pepper to taste

Method:

1. Add all ingredients to a bowl.
2. Mix well.
3. Transfer to a slow cooker.
4. Cover the pot.
5. Cook for 8 hours on low.
6. Discard bay leaves.
7. Let cool.
8. Transfer to food containers.
9. Freeze for up to 1 month.
10. Reheat before serving.

Nutritional Content:

- Calories: 270
- Fat: 8 g
- Cholesterol: 20 mg
- Sodium: 151 mg

- Carbohydrates: 12 g
- Fiber: 2 g
- Sugars: 7 g
- Protein: 45 g

Asian-Style Pork Tenderloin

Preparation Time: 2 hours and 10 minutes
Cooking Time: 6 hours
Servings: 8

Ingredients:

Marinade

- 4 cloves garlic, minced
- 1 tablespoon ginger
- ¼ cup brown sugar
- ¼ cup reduced-sodium soy sauce
- 2 tablespoons rice vinegar
- 2 tablespoons lemon juice
- 1 tablespoon dry mustard
- 2 tablespoons Worcestershire sauce
- Pepper to taste

Pork

- 2 lb. pork tenderloin sliced into thin strips

Method:

1. Add all marinade ingredients to a bowl.
2. Mix well.
3. Soak the pork in the marinade.
4. Cover and refrigerate for 2 hours or transfer to sealable plastic bags and freeze for up to 2 months.
5. When ready to cook, cook in the slow cooker for 6 hours.

Nutritional Content:

- Calories: 256
- Fat: 9g
- Cholesterol: 5mg
- Carbohydrates: 9g
- Fiber: 0g
- Sugars: 8g
- Sodium: 658 mg
- Protein: 34g

Greek Chicken

Preparation Time: 15 minutes
Cooking Time: 45 minutes
Servings: 4

Ingredients:

- 1 teaspoon garlic powder
- ½ cup Parmesan cheese, grated
- 1 cup plain Greek yogurt
- Salt and pepper to taste
- Cooking spray
- 4 chicken breast fillets

Method:

1. Preheat your oven to 375 degrees.
2. In a bowl, mix the garlic powder, Parmesan cheese, yogurt, salt and pepper.
3. Cover your baking pan with foil.
4. Spray it with foil.
5. Spread yogurt mixture on both sides of chicken.
6. Add to the baking pan.
7. Bake for 45 minutes.
8. Let cool.
9. Transfer to food containers.
10. Refrigerate for up to 2 days.
11. Serve with steamed vegetables.

Nutritional Content:

- Calories: 266
- Fat: 4g
- Cholesterol: 3mg
- Carbohydrates: 3g
- Dietary Fiber: 0g
- Sugars: 2g
- Protein: 46g

Tofu & Quinoa Bowl

Preparation Time: 30 minutes
Cooking Time: 40 minutes
Servings: 6

Ingredients:

- 15 oz. tofu, sliced into cubes
- 1 tablespoon sesame oil
- 1 tablespoon reduced-sodium soy sauce
- 6 cups cooked quinoa
- 1 cup carrots, shredded
- ½ cup cilantro, chopped
- ¼ cup scallions, chopped
- ½ cup slivered almonds

Sauce

- 1 clove garlic, minced
- 1 teaspoon ginger, grated
- 2 teaspoons peanut butter
- 3 tablespoons coconut milk
- 2 tablespoons rice wine vinegar
- 2 tablespoons hot sauce
- ½ tablespoon brown sugar
- 1 tablespoon lime juice

Method:

1. Preheat your oven to 350 degrees F.
2. In a bowl, toss the tofu in oil and soy sauce.
3. Spread tofu in your baking pan.
4. Bake for 40 minutes.
5. Add tofu, quinoa, carrots, cilantro, scallions and almonds to food containers.
6. Refrigerate for up to 2 days.
7. Reheat before serving.
8. In a bowl, mix the sauce ingredients.
9. Transfer to a sauce cup and refrigerate until ready to serve.

10. Reheat before drizzling on top of the tofu, quinoa and veggies.

Nutritional Content:

- Calories: 232
- Fat: 10 g
- Cholesterol: 0 mg
- Carbohydrates: 27 g
- Fiber: 4.5 g
- Sugars: 4 g
- Protein: 12 g

Crispy Tuna Patties

Preparation Time: 15 minutes
Cooking Time: 6 minutes
Servings: 8

Ingredients:

- 12 oz. canned tuna flakes
- 4 egg whites
- 16 wheat crackers, crushed
- ¼ cup carrot, grated
- ¼ cup capers, diced
- 1 tablespoon onion, minced
- Dried mustard to taste
- Cooking spray

Method:

1. Combine ingredients in a bowl.
2. Form patties from the mixture.
3. Wrap patties with cling wrap or foil.
4. Freeze for up to 1 month.
5. When ready to cook, spray your pan with oil.
6. Place it over medium heat.
7. Cook patties for 3 minutes per side.
8. Serve immediately.

Nutritional Content:

- Calories: 80 calories
- Fat: 1 gram
- Cholesterol: 22 g
- Carbohydrate: 4 g
- Sodium: 240 mg
- Sugar: 0 g
- Protein: 12 g

Baked Chicken & Vegetables

Preparation Time: 20 minutes
Cooking Time: 1 hour
Servings: 6

Ingredients:

- 1 onion, sliced into wedges
- 6 carrots, sliced
- 4 potatoes, sliced
- 6 chicken breast fillets, sliced into cubes
- 1 teaspoon thyme
- Pepper to taste
- ½ cup water

Method:

1. Preheat your oven to 400 degrees F.
2. Toss onion, carrots and potatoes in a baking pan.
3. Arrange chicken on top.
4. In a bowl, combine thyme, pepper and water.
5. Pour on top of the chicken.
6. Bake in the oven for 1 hour.
7. Let cool.
8. Transfer to food container.
9. Refrigerate for up to 2 days.
10. Reheat before serving.

Nutritional Content:

- Calories: 240
- Cholesterol: 13mg
- Carbohydrate: 25 g
- Sugar: 10 g
- Fat: 3.5 g
- Sodium: 130 mg
- Fiber: 4 g
- Protein: 26 g

Pork & Black Bean Stew

Preparation Time: 10 minutes
Cooking Time: 1 hour and 15 minutes
Servings: 4

Ingredients:

- 2 teaspoons olive oil
- 1 lb. lean pork loin or tenderloin, sliced into cubes
- 1 cup onion, chopped
- 3 cloves garlic, minced
- 2 cups canned chipotle peppers in adobo sauce, minced
- Garlic powder to taste
- 1 teaspoon ground cumin
- 14 oz. unsalted chicken broth
- 14 oz. low-sodium canned black beans, rinsed and drained
- 14 oz. low-sodium canned diced tomatoes

Method:

1. Add oil to a pan over medium high heat.
2. Cook pork cubes until golden on all sides.
3. Add onion, garlic, chipotle peppers, garlic powder and cumin.
4. Cook for 2 to 3 minutes, stirring.
5. Pour in broth, beans and tomatoes.
6. Bring to a boil.
7. Reduce heat and simmer for 1 hour.

Nutritional Content:

- Calories: 308
- Fat: 7 g
- Cholesterol: 84 mg
- Carbohydrate: 25 g
- Sodium: 414 mg
- Fiber: 6 g
- Protein: 33 g

Sweet & Sour Pork

Preparation Time: 15 minutes
Cooking Time: 40 minutes
Servings: 6

Ingredients:

- Cooking spray
- 1 lb. lean pork tenderloin, sliced into strips
- ¼ cup pineapple juice
- ¼ cup Splenda sweetener
- ½ cup water
- 2 tablespoons cornstarch
- 1 tablespoon reduced-sodium soy sauce
- Salt to taste
- 1 onion, sliced
- 1 red bell pepper, sliced
- 15 oz. pineapple chunks
- ¼ cup rice vinegar

Method:

1. Spray your pan with oil.
2. Place it over medium high heat.
3. Cook pork until golden on both sides.
4. Transfer to a plate.
5. Remove fat from the pan.
6. In a bowl, mix the pineapple juice, sweetener, water, cornstarch, soy sauce and salt.
7. Add to the pan.
8. Cook for 2 minutes.
9. Put pork back to the pan.
10. Cook for 30 minutes.
11. Add remaining ingredients.
12. Cook for 5 minutes.

Nutritional Content:

- Calories: 248
- Fat: 3.5 g

- Cholesterol: 60 mg
- Carbohydrate: 36 g
- Sodium: 354 mg

- Sugar: 8 g
- Protein: 18 g

Creamy Chicken

Preparation Time: 20 minutes
Cooking Time: 4 hours
Servings: 6

Ingredients:

- Cooking spray
- 6 chicken breast fillets
- ½ cup chicken stock
- 11 oz. low-fat cream of mushroom soup
- 1 cup plain Greek yogurt
- 8 oz. mushrooms
- 1 packet Italian dressing mix

Method:

1. Spray your pan with oil.
2. Place it over medium heat.
3. Cook chicken until brown on both sides.
4. Transfer to a slow cooker.
5. Stir in the rest of the ingredients.
6. Cover the pot.
7. Cook on low for 4 hours.

Nutritional Content:

- Calories: 128
- Fat: 1.68 g
- Cholesterol: 90mg
- Sugar: 2.28 g
- Sodium: 257mg
- ·Protein: 18.5 g

Chicken Casserole

Preparation Time: 30 minutes
Cooking Time: 30 minutes
Servings: 4

Ingredients:

- 2 cups frozen mixed veggies
- 1 cup whole wheat pasta, cooked
- 1 cup chicken breast, cooked and sliced into cubes
- 10 ½ oz. nonfat cream of chicken soup
- 1 cup low-fat cheddar cheese, shredded
- 4 oz. mushrooms
- ¾ cup water
- Onion powder to taste

Method:

1. Spray your casserole dish with oil.
2. In a pan over medium heat, cook frozen veggies according to directions.
3. In a bowl, mix cooked veggies, cooked pasta and remaining ingredients.
4. Pour mixture into a casserole dish.
5. Cover and refrigerate for up to 1 day.
6. When ready to cook, bake in the oven at 350 degrees F for 30 minutes.

Nutritional Content:

- Calories: 256
- Fat: 8 g
- Cholesterol: 12 mg
- Carbohydrate: 27 g
- Sodium: 834 mg
- Sugar: 3 g
- Protein: 19 g

Ginger Beef Stir Fry

Preparation Time: 15 minutes
Cooking Time: 10 minutes
Servings: 6

Ingredients:

- 1 lb. flank steak, sliced into strips
- 2 cloves garlic, minced
- 2 teaspoons ground ginger
- 6 oz. nonfat beef broth
- 1 tablespoons cornstarch
- 3 tablespoons low-sodium soy sauce
- ¼ cup hoisin sauce
- 1 teaspoon canola oil
- ¼ teaspoon red pepper flakes
- 1 red bell pepper, sliced into strips
- 3 oz. broccoli florets

Method:

1. Season steak with garlic and ginger. Set aside.
2. In a bowl, mix broth, cornstarch, soy sauce and hoisin sauce. Mix well.
3. Pour oil into a pan over medium heat.
4. Add red pepper flakes.
5. Cook beef strips for 5 minutes, stirring often.
6. Add bell pepper and broccoli.
7. Cook for 2 minutes.
8. Add broth mixture.
9. Cook for 2 minutes.
10. Let cool.
11. Transfer to food containers.
12. Refrigerate for up to 3 days.
13. Reheat before serving.
14. Serve with brown rice.

Nutritional Content:

- Calories: 275
- Fat: 8 g
- Carbohydrates: 25 g

- Dietary Fiber: 2 g
- Sugars: 6 g
- Protein: 17 g

Cajun Chicken

Preparation Time: 30 minutes
Cooking Time: 1 hour
Servings: 4

Ingredients:

- 1 lb. chicken breast fillets
- 1 cup spinach, cooked and drained
- 3 oz. low-fat pepper Jack cheese, shredded
- 1 tablespoon breadcrumbs
- 2 tablespoons Cajun seasoning
- 2 teaspoons olive oil

Method:

1. Flatten chicken with a meat mallet.
2. In a bowl, mix spinach and cheese.
3. In another bowl, mix breadcrumbs and seasoning.
4. Spread spinach mixture on top of chicken breast and roll them up.
5. Brush chicken with oil and coat with seasoned breadcrumbs.
6. Wrap each rolled chicken with foil or plastic wrap.
7. Freeze for up to 1 week.
8. When ready to cook, place in a baking pan.
9. Bake at 350 degrees F for 50 minutes to 1 hour.

Nutritional Content:

- Calories: 241
- Fat: 9.7g
- Carbohydrates: 2g
- Dietary Fiber: 1g
- Sugars: 0g
- Protein: 32g

Barbecue Salmon

Preparation Time: 15 minutes
Cooking Time: 15 minutes
Servings: 4

Ingredients:

- 2 tablespoons lemon juice
- ¼ cup pineapple juice
- 4 salmon fillets
- 4 teaspoons chili powder
- 2 tablespoons brown sugar
- ¾ teaspoon ground cumin
- 2 teaspoons lemon zest
- ¼ teaspoon cinnamon

Method:

1. Preheat your oven to 400 degrees.
2. Mix lemon juice and pineapple juice in a sealable plastic bag.
3. Add salmon fillets.
4. Chill in the refrigerator for 1 hour.
5. Mix remaining ingredients.
6. Sprinkle fish with the mixture.
7. Bake in the oven for 15 minutes.
8. Transfer to food container and refrigerate for up to 3 days.
9. Reheat in the oven before serving.

Nutritional Content:

- Calories: 225
- Fat: 6 g
- Cholesterol: 88 mg
- Carbohydrate: 7 g
- Sodium: 407 mg
- Sugar: 6 g
- Protein: 34 g

Crispy Chicken

Preparation Time: 1 hour and 20 minutes
Cooking Time: 30 minutes
Servings: 3

Ingredients:

- ¼ cup low-fat buttermilk
- ⅛ tsp. paprika
- 12 oz. chicken breast tenders
- ¼ cup bran cereal
- 1 tablespoon dry onion soup mix
- ¼ cup panko breadcrumbs

Method:

1. Mix milk and paprika in a bowl.
2. Put chicken in the bowl.
3. Coat with the mixture.
4. Cover and refrigerate for 1 hour.
5. Add cereal to a food processor.
6. Pulse until fully ground.
7. Mix ground cereal with onion soup mix and breadcrumbs.
8. Coat chicken with the breadcrumb mixture.
9. Place in a food container.
10. Freeze for up to 2 weeks.
11. When ready to cook, bake in the oven at 375 degrees F for 15 minutes per side.

Nutritional Content:

- Calories: 210
- Fat: 3.5g
- Cholesterol: 2 mg
- Carbohydrates: 17g
- Fiber: 3.5g
- Sugar: 2g
- Protein: 29g

Chapter 7: Snacks

Chicken & Cheese Steak Wrap

Preparation Time: 10 minutes
Cooking Time: 7 minutes
Serving: 1

Ingredients:

- Cooking spray
- ¼ cup onion, chopped
- ¼ lb. chicken breast fillet, sliced into thin strips
- ¼ cup green bell pepper, chopped
- ¼ cup mushrooms, sliced
- ¾ cup Swiss cheese
- 1 whole wheat flour

Method:

1. Spray your pan with oil.
2. Add onion and chicken.
3. Cook for 3 to 5 minutes.
4. Stir in bell pepper and mushrooms for 2 minutes.
5. Let cool.
6. Transfer to food container.
7. When ready to serve, reheat mixture.
8. Add mixture and cheese on top of the tortilla.
9. Roll up and serve.

Nutritional Content:

- Calories: 264
- Carbohydrate: 17 g
- Fat: 6 g
- Protein: 33 g
- Cholesterol: 76 mg
- Sodium: 620 mg
- Fiber: 4 g

Chicken Rolls

Preparation Time: 30 minutes
Cooking Time: 30 minutes
Servings: 8

Ingredients:

- 8 chicken breasts, sliced into cubes
- ½ cup Italian seasoned breadcrumbs
- ¼ cup parmesan cheese, grated
- 6 tablespoons egg whites
- 5 oz. spinach, cooked
- 6 tablespoons ricotta cheese
- 6 oz. low-fat and unsalted mozzarella, shredded
- 1 cup marinara sauce

Method:

1. Sprinkle chicken with salt and pepper.
2. In a bowl, mix breadcrumbs with Parmesan cheese.
3. Add egg whites to another bowl.
4. In another bowl, mix mozzarella with spinach and ricotta cheese.
5. Top each chicken with the mozzarella mixture.
6. Roll them up.
7. Soak in egg whites and coat with breadcrumbs.
8. Arrange in a single layer in a food container.
9. Freeze for up to 1 month.
10. When ready to cook, bake in the oven at 450 degrees for 20 to 30 minutes.
11. Top with marinara sauce and serve.

Nutritional Content:

- Calories: 268
- Fat: 9 g
- Cholesterol: 0 mg
- Carbohydrates: 8 g
- Fiber: 1.5 g
- Sugars: 3 g
- Protein: 36 g

Turkey Turnover

Preparation Time: 10 minutes
Cooking Time: 15 minutes
Servings: 24

Ingredients:

- 1 cup low-fat cheese, shredded
- 1 lb. ground turkey
- 1 packet dry onion soup
- 3 tubes low-fat refrigerated crescent rolls

Method:

1. Combine cheese, ground turkey and onion soup mix in a pan over medium heat.
2. Separate rolls and slice in triangle.
3. Spread mixture on top of the triangles.
4. Fold over and seal the edges.
5. Freeze until ready to serve.
6. When ready to cook, bake in the oven at 350 degrees F for 15 minutes.

Nutritional Content:

- Calories: 155
- Fat: 7 g
- Cholesterol: 14 mg
- Carbohydrate: 13 g
- Sodium: 472 mg
- Sugar: 3 g
- Protein: 9 g

Stuffed French Toast

Preparation Time: 10 minutes
Cooking Time: 5 minutes
Servings: 1

Ingredients:

- ½ cup ricotta cheese
- 4 slices bread
- 2 packets sugar substitute
- 3 egg whites, beaten
- ¼ teaspoon vanilla extract
- ¼ teaspoon pumpkin pie spice
- Cooking spray

Method:

1. Spread ricotta on top of 2 bread slices.
2. Sprinkle with sugar
3. Add 2 bread slices on top to make sandwich.
4. Mix egg white, vanilla extract and pumpkin pie spice.
5. Dip bread in egg white mixture.
6. Freeze until ready to cook.
7. When ready to cook, fry in a pan misted with oil until golden.

Nutritional Content:

- Calories: 227
- Fat: .5 g
- Cholesterol: 20 mg
- Carbohydrate: 27 g
- Sodium: 659 mg
- Sugar: 8 g
- Protein: 25 g

Veggie Pizza

Preparation Time: 20 minutes
Cooking Time: 20 minutes
Servings: 8

Ingredients:

- ¼ cup dry ranch dressing mix
- ½ cup light sour cream
- ½ cup low-fat onion and chive cream cheese
- 2 low-carb tortilla wraps
- ¾ cup tomatoes, diced
- ¾ cup broccoli florets
- ⅛ cup green bell pepper, diced
- ⅛ cup carrots, shredded
- ⅛ cup cucumbers, diced
- ½ cup black olives, sliced
- ¾ cup Monterey Jack cheese, shredded

Method:

1. Combine ranch dressing mix, sour cream and cream cheese.
2. Spread mixture on top of tortillas.
3. Top with vegetables and cheese.
4. Cover with foil or plastic wrap.
5. Freeze for up to 1 week.
6. When ready to cook, bake in the oven at 350 degrees F for 20 minutes.

Nutritional Content:

- Calories: 170
- Fat: 10 g
- Protein: 10 g
- Carbohydrate: 12 g
- Cholesterol: 23 mg
- Sodium: 870 mg
- Sugar: 1.6 g
- Fiber: 4 g

Chicken Caprese

Preparation Time: 5 minutes
Cooking Time: 6 minutes
Servings: 4

Ingredients:

- 1 lb. chicken breast fillet
- 1 tablespoon olive oil
- Pepper to taste
- 1 teaspoon Italian seasoning
- 1 tomato, sliced thickly
- 4 mozzarella cheese slices
- 3 tablespoons balsamic vinegar
- 2 tablespoons basil, sliced thinly

Method:

1. Drizzle chicken with oil.
2. Season with pepper and Italian seasoning.
3. Heat a grill or grill pan over medium high heat.
4. Grill chicken for 3 minutes per side.
5. Let cool.
6. Transfer to food containers.
7. When ready to serve, reheat on the grill.
8. Top with the remaining ingredients and serve.

Nutritional Content:

- Calories: 230
- Fat: 9 gram
- Cholesterol: 80 mg
- Sodium: 105 mg
- Carbohydrates: 4 g
- Dietary Fiber: 0 g
- Sugar: 2.5 g
- Protein: 33 g

Chicken Wrap

Preparation Time: 15 minutes
Cooking Time: 15 minutes
Servings: 4

Ingredients:

Sauce

- 8 oz. water chestnuts, minced
- 8 oz. bamboo shoots, minced
- 2 tablespoons hoisin sauce
- 3 tablespoons sherry cooking wine
- 2 packets Splenda sweetener
- 2 teaspoons reduced-sodium soy sauce
- 1 tablespoon no-salt peanut butter
- 2 teaspoons hot pepper sauce

Chicken

- 1 teaspoon olive oil
- 1 tablespoon garlic, minced
- 1 cup onion, minced
- 1 teaspoon ginger, minced
- ½ lb. ground chicken breast
- 8 large lettuce leaves
- 1 cucumber, sliced into strips

Method:

1. Mix sauce ingredients in a bowl. Set aside.
2. Add oil to a pan over medium heat.
3. Cook onion and garlic for 5 minutes.
4. Add ginger and chicken.
5. Cook for 4 minutes.
6. Stir in sauce mixture.
7. Cook for 2 to 4 minutes.
8. Turn off heat.
9. Let cool.

10. Transfer to food containers.
11. Refrigerate for up to 2 days.
12. When ready to serve, reheat mixture.
13. Top lettuce with the mixture and with cucumber strips.
14. Roll them up and serve.

Nutritional Content:

- Calories: 155
- Fat: 4 g
- Cholesterol: 33 mg
- Carbohydrates: 11 g

- Sodium: 637 mg
- Dietary Fiber: 5 g
- Sugar: 4 g
- Protein: 16 g

Zucchini Boats

Preparation Time: 20 minutes
Cooking Time: 30 minutes
Servings: 8

Ingredients:

- 4 zucchinis, sliced in half and flesh scooped out
- 1 lb. ground turkey breast
- ½ white onion, chopped
- 1 egg, beaten
- 1 tomato, diced
- ½ lb. mushrooms, sliced
- ¼ cup whole wheat breadcrumbs
- ¾ cup spaghetti sauce
- Salt and pepper to taste
- 1 cup low fat mozzarella cheese, shredded

Method:

1. Microwave zucchini halves for 3 minutes.
2. Drain. Set aside.
3. In a pan over medium heat, cook onion and ground turkey for 3 to 5 minutes.
4. In a bowl, mix turkey mixture with the rest of the ingredients except cheese.
5. Spread mixture on top of zucchini boats.
6. Top with cheese.
7. Cover with foil and refrigerate for up to 1 day.
8. When ready to cook, bake in the oven at 350 degrees F for 20 minutes.

Nutritional Content:

- Calories: 195
- Fat: 7.5g
- Cholesterol: 0 mg
- Sodium: 294 mg
- Carbohydrates: 16g
- Fiber: 4g
- Sugars: 5g
- Protein: 17.5g

Stuffed Acorn Squash

Preparation Time: 10 minutes
Cooking Time: 20 minutes
Servings: 4

Ingredients:

- 2 acorn squash, sliced in half and seeds removed
- 1 cup onion, chopped
- 1 cup celery, diced
- 1 cup mushrooms, sliced
- 1 lb. lean ground turkey
- 1 teaspoon basil
- 1 teaspoon oregano
- 1 teaspoon garlic powder
- Salt and pepper to taste
- 8 oz. canned tomato sauce
- 1 cup low-fat cheddar cheese, shredded

Method:

1. Preheat your oven to 350 degrees F.
2. Bake the squash in the oven for 40 minutes.
3. In a pan over medium heat, cook onion, celery, mushrooms and turkey for 5 minutes.
4. Season with herbs, spices, salt and pepper.
5. Add tomato sauce.
6. Refrigerate squash and sauce mixture in separate containers.
7. When ready to cook, top squash with sauce mixture and cheese.
8. Bake in the oven at 350 degrees F for 15 minutes.

Nutritional Content:

- Calories: 299
- Fat: 4 g
- Carbohydrates: 38g
- Fiber: 6g
- Sugars: 9g
- Protein: 30g

Pesto Pasta

Preparation Time: 15 minutes
Cooking Time: 0 minute
Servings: 4

Ingredients:

- 1 tablespoon olive oil
- ½ cup water
- ¼ cup fresh basil leaves
- 2 cloves garlic, minced
- 10 oz. spinach, chopped
- 2 tablespoons Parmesan cheese, grated
- 4 cups cooked whole wheat pasta

Method:

1. Add all ingredients except to a food processor.
2. Pulse until smooth.
3. Refrigerate pesto sauce for up to 5 days.
4. When ready to serve, toss cooked pasta in sauce and serve.

Nutritional Content:

- Calories: 77
- Fat: 5 g
- Cholesterol: 3 mg
- Carbohydrate: 4 gram
- Sodium: 292 mg
- Sugar: 1 gram
- Protein: 6 g

Chapter 8: Desserts

Pumpkin Mousse

Preparation Time: 5 minutes
Cooking Time: 0 minute
Servings: 4

Ingredients:

- 15 oz. pumpkin puree
- 2 cups whipped topping (sugar free)
- ½ cup skim milk
- 1 teaspoon cinnamon
- Pinch nutmeg

Method:

1. In a bowl, combine all ingredients.
2. Mix until creamy.
3. Transfer to glass jars with lids.
4. Refrigerate for up to 3 days.

Nutritional Content:

- Calories: 149
- Fat: 4.4 g
- Protein: 2 g
- Carbohydrate: 28 g
- Cholesterol: 0 mg
- Sodium: 71 mg
- Sugar: 8.6 g
- Fiber: 3.4 g

Brownie Bites

Preparation Time: 15 minutes
Cooking Time: 10 minutes
Servings: 4

Ingredients:

- 2 eggs
- 1 avocado, sliced
- 3 tablespoons butter
- ½ Splenda
- ½ teaspoon vanilla extract
- ¼ cup dark chocolate chips
- ½ cup cocoa powder
- ½ teaspoon salt
- ½ cup almond flour
- 1 teaspoon baking soda

Method:

1. Preheat your oven to 350 degrees F.
2. Add eggs, avocado, butter, Splenda and vanilla extract to a food processor.
3. Pulse until smooth.
4. Transfer to a bowl.
5. Add the remaining ingredients.
6. Pour mixture into a muffin pan.
7. Bake in the oven for 10 minutes.
8. Let cool.
9. Transfer to airtight container.
10. Refrigerate for up to 1 week.

Nutritional Content:

- Calories: 150
- Fat: 5 g
- Cholesterol: 0 mg
- Sodium: 15 mg
- Carbohydrates: 22 g
- Fiber: 3 g
- Sugar: 4 g
- Protein: 6 g

Jello

Preparation Time: 5 minutes
Cooking Time: 0 minute
Servings: 4

Ingredients:

- 1 box jello (sugar-free)
- 8 tablespoons whipped topping (sugar free)

Method:

1. Follow package directions for making jello.
2. Refrigerate until set.
3. Divide jello into 4 glass jars with lid.
4. Top with the whipped topping.
5. Refrigerate for up to 3 days.

Nutritional Content:

- Calories: 30
- Fat: 0 g
- Cholesterol: 0 mg
- Carbohydrate: 2 g
- Sodium: 65 mg
- Sugar: 1 g
- Protein: 1 gram

Dessert Cups

Preparation Time: 5 minutes
Cooking Time: 3 minutes
Servings: 18

Ingredients:

- ¼ teaspoon coconut oil, melted
- ½ cup coconut butter, softened
- 2 cups chocolate chips (sugar free)

Method:

1. Line your muffin tin with liners.
2. Mix all ingredients in a bowl.
3. Pour mixture into muffin cups.
4. Freeze until ready to serve.

Nutritional Content:

- Calories: 120
- Fat: 8 g
- Cholesterol: 10 mg
- Sodium: 1 mg
- Carbohydrates: 6 g
- Fiber: 4 g
- Sugar: 1 g
- Protein: 1 g

Chocolate Mousse

Preparation Time: 5 minutes
Cooking Time: 0 minute
Servings: 4

Ingredients:

- 1/8 cup cocoa powder
- 4 oz. cream cheese (fat free)
- 2 tablespoons almond milk (unsweetened)
- 1 teaspoon vanilla extract
- ¼ cup honey
- ¾ cup light whipped topping

Method:

1. Use a hand mixer to mix ingredients except whipped topping.
2. Stir in the whipped topping.
3. Transfer to glass jars with lid.
4. Refrigerate until ready to serve or for up to 3 days.

Nutritional Content:

- Calories: 63
- Fat: 2 g
- Cholesterol: 10 mg
- Sodium: 102 mg
- Carbohydrates: 7 g
- Fiber: 3 g
- Sugar: 2 g
- Protein: 4 g

Cheesecake Pudding

Preparation Time: 5 minutes
Cooking Time: 0 minute
Servings: 1

Ingredients:

- 1 cup nonfat plain Greek yogurt
- 1 package cheesecake pudding mix (sugar-free)

Method:

1. Add yogurt and pudding mix to a food processor.
2. Pulse until smooth.
3. Transfer to food containers.
4. Refrigerate for up to 3 days.

Nutritional Content:

- Calories: 31
- Carbohydrate: 5 g
- Fat: 2 g (0 g saturated)
- Protein: 6 g
- Cholesterol: 1 mg
- Sodium: 105 mg
- Fiber: 0 g

Silky Fudge Dessert

Preparation Time: 40 minutes
Cooking Time: 0 minute
Servings: 8

Ingredients:

- 1 packed unflavored gelatin
- ¼ cup hot water
- 1.4 oz. instant pudding mix (sugar and fat free)
- 1 cup cold skim milk
- 16 oz. silken tofu, diced
- ½ teaspoon vanilla extract

Method:

1. Combine gelatin and hot water.
2. Let the mixture become firm.
3. In another bowl, blend the pudding mix and milk.
4. Add tofu to the pudding mixture.
5. Stir in vanilla extract.
6. Add tofu mixture to a food processor.
7. Pulse until smooth.
8. Add gelatin and stir.
9. Pour into a baking pan.
10. Refrigerate for 30 minutes.
11. Transfer to food containers and refrigerate for up to 3 days.

Nutritional Content:

- Calories: 56
- Fat: 1 g
- Cholesterol: 1 mg
- Carbohydrate: 6 g
- Sodium: 181 mg
- Fiber: 0 g
- Protein: 5 g

Cream Cheese Cookies

Preparation Time: 10 minutes
Cooking Time: 15 minutes
Servings: 24

Ingredients:

- 3 cups almond flour
- 2 oz. cream cheese
- ¼ cup butter, softened
- 1 egg, beaten
- 1/3 cup monk fruit blend
- 2 teaspoons vanilla extract
- 1 teaspoon Splenda
- Pinch salt

Method:

1. Combine all ingredients in a bowl.
2. Form cookies from the mixture.
3. Bake at 350 degrees for 15 minutes.
4. Let cool.
5. Transfer to airtight container.
6. Refrigerate for up to 1 week.

Nutritional Content:

- Calories: 110
- Fat: 10g
- Cholesterol: 10mg
- Carbohydrate: 3g
- Fiber: 2g
- Sugar: 1g
- Protein: 3g

Spinach & Strawberry Salad

Preparation Time: 10 minutes
Cooking Time: 0 minute
Servings: 4

Ingredients:

- 10 oz. spinach, sliced
- 1 qt. strawberries, sliced
- ¼ cup almonds, slivered

Dressing

- ½ cup olive oil
- ¼ cup white vinegar
- 1 tablespoon onion, minced
- 1 tablespoon poppy seeds
- 2 tablespoons sesame seeds
- ¼ teaspoon Worcestershire sauce
- ¼ teaspoon paprika

Method:

1. Arrange spinach in food containers.
2. Top with strawberries and almonds.
3. Mix dressing ingredients in a glass jar with lid.
4. Shake to blend well.
5. Refrigerate salad and dressing for up to 2 days.
6. Pour dressing over salad when ready to serve.

Nutritional Content:

- Calories: 490
- Fat: 35.2

Pudding Bites

Preparation Time: 5 minutes
Cooking Time: 5 minutes
Servings: 1

Ingredients:

- 2 tablespoons Splenda
- 1 cup skim milk
- 3 cups low-sugar chocolate chips
- ½ teaspoon vanilla extract

Method:

1. Mix the Splenda and milk in a pan over medium heat.
2. Cook while stirring for 1 minute.
3. Stir in the baking chips.
4. Add vanilla extract and turn off heat.
5. Transfer to glass jars with lid.
6. Refrigerate until ready to serve or for up to 3 days.

Nutritional Content:

- Calories: 142
- Fat: 7.2 g
- Cholesterol: 0 mg
- Sodium: 0 mg
- Carbohydrates: 20.4 g
- Fiber: 0 g
- Sugar: 6.4 g
- Protein: 5.6 g

Chocolate Chip Cookies

Preparation Time: 10 minutes
Cooking Time: 12 minutes
Servings: 12

Ingredients:

- ½ cup butter, melted
- ¾ cup Splenda
- 1 egg, beaten
- 1 teaspoon vanilla extract
- 1 ½ cups almond flour
- ¼ teaspoon salt
- ½ teaspoon baking powder
- ¾ cup chocolate chips (sugar-free)

Method:

1. Preheat your oven to 350 degrees F.
2. Mix butter and Splenda in a bowl.
3. Stir in egg and vanilla.
4. Add the remaining ingredients.
5. Mix well.
6. Form cookies from the mixture.
7. Bake in the oven for 10 to 12 minutes.
8. Let cool.
9. Transfer to airtight container.
10. Refrigerate for up to 1 week.

Nutritional Content:

- Calories: 135
- Fat: 6 g
- Cholesterol: 3 mg
- Sodium: 27 mg
- Carbohydrates: 20 g
- Fiber: 2 g
- Sugar: 2 g
- Protein: 5 g

Chapter 9: Salads

Carrot & Cucumber Salad

Preparation Time: 15 minutes
Cooking Time: 0 minute
Servings: 2

Ingredients:

- 1 cup carrot, sliced
- ½ cucumber, sliced
- 2 tablespoons red bell pepper, minced
- 2 tablespoons green onion, chopped

Dressing

- ¼ cup rice vinegar
- 1 teaspoon Splenda
- ½ teaspoon olive oil
- ¼ teaspoon ginger, grated

Method:

1. Toss carrot, cucumber, red bell pepper and green onion in food containers.
2. Seal. Refrigerate for up to 2 days.
3. Mix dressing ingredients.
4. Store in glass jar with lid.
5. Refrigerate.
6. Pour dressing over salad when ready to serve.

Nutritional Content:

- Calories: 58
- Fat: 1.4 g
- Cholesterol: 0 mg
- Sodium: 35 mg
- Carbohydrates: 11 g
- Fiber: 2.4 g
- Sugar: 3 g
- Protein: 1.4 g

Summer Salad

Preparation Time: 15 minutes
Cooking Time: 0 minute
Servings: 4

Ingredients:

- 4 cups Romaine lettuce
- 1 apple, diced
- 1 pear, diced
- ¼ cup dried cranberries
- ¼ cup Swiss cheese, shredded
- ¼ cup cashews

Dressing

- ¼ cup olive oil
- ¼ cup orange juice
- 1 teaspoon onion, minced
- 1 tablespoon Splenda
- 1 tablespoon poppy seeds
- Pinch salt

Method:

1. Arrange Romaine lettuce in food containers.
2. Sprinkle fruits, cheese and cashews on top.
3. Seal the food container.
4. Refrigerate for up to 1 day.
5. Mix dressing ingredients in a sauce cup or glass jar with lid.
6. Drizzle salad with dressing when ready to serve.

Nutritional Content:

- Calories: 314
- Fat: 24.4 g
- Cholesterol: 9 mg
- Sodium: 342 mg
- Carbohydrates: 21.3 g
- Fiber: 1.8 g
- Sugar: 4 g
- Protein: 5.5 g

Cucumber Salad

Preparation Time: 10 minutes
Cooking Time: 0 minute
Servings: 4

Ingredients:

- 1 white onion, chopped
- 4 cucumbers, sliced thinly
- ½ cup water
- 1 cup white vinegar
- 2 tablespoons dried dill
- 1 tablespoon cup Splenda

Method:

1. Combine all ingredients in a bowl.
2. Divide into 4 food containers
3. Seal and refrigerate for up to 3 days.

Nutritional Content:

- Calories: 98
- Fat: 0.2 g
- Cholesterol: 0 mg
- Sodium: 4.4 mg
- Carbohydrates: 20 g
- Fiber: 1 g
- Sugar: 2 g
- Protein: 1 g

Green Salad

Preparation Time: 10 minutes
Cooking Time: 0 minute
Servings: 4

Ingredients:

Salad

- 4 cups mixed salad greens
- 1 avocado, sliced into cubes
- ½ cup almonds, sliced

Dressing

- 4 tablespoons olive oil
- 1 tablespoon Dijon mustard
- 2 cloves garlic, minced
- 1 teaspoon fresh parsley, chopped
- 1/8 teaspoon Splenda
- 2 tablespoons white wine vinegar
- 1 teaspoon lemon juice
- Salt and pepper to taste

Method:

1. Arrange salad greens in food containers.
2. Top with avocado and almonds.
3. Seal and refrigerate for up to 3 days.
4. Combine dressing in a separate container.
5. Refrigerate until ready to serve.
6. Drizzle with dressing before serving.

Nutritional Content:

- Calories: 325
- Fat: 15 g
- Cholesterol: 12.6 mg
- Sodium: 561 mg
- Carbohydrates: 10.5 g
- Fiber: 5.9 g
- Sugar: 1.8 g
- Protein: 6.5 g

Roasted Beet Salad

Preparation Time: 10 minutes
Cooking Time: 50 minutes
Servings: 4

Ingredients:

- 2 beets, trimmed
- 2 tablespoons balsamic vinegar
- 2 teaspoons maple syrup
- Salt and pepper to taste

Method:

1. Preheat your oven to 400 degrees F.
2. Wrap beets with foil.
3. Add to a baking pan.
4. Roast in the oven for 50 minutes.
5. Unwrap and let cool. Peel and slice the beets.
6. Mix remaining ingredients in a bowl.
7. Pour mixture over the beets.
8. Transfer to food containers.
9. Refrigerate for up to 2 days.

Nutritional Content:

- Calories: 66
- Fat: 0.2 g
- Cholesterol: 0 mg
- Sodium: 135 mg
- Carbohydrates: 15 g
- Fiber: 3.4 g
- Sugar: 4 g
- Protein: 2 g

Spinach & Cranberry Salad

Preparation Time: 10 minutes
Cooking Time: 0 minute
Servings: 8

Ingredients:

- 1 lb. spinach, sliced
- 1 cup dried cranberries
- 2 tablespoons toasted sesame seeds
- ¾ cup almonds, slivered
- 1 tablespoon poppy seeds

Dressing

- ½ cup cider vinegar
- ½ cup olive oil
- 2 teaspoons onion, minced
- ¼ teaspoon paprika

Method:

1. Toss spinach and cranberries in food containers.
2. Top with the sesame seeds, almond and poppy seeds.
3. In a separate container, mix dressing ingredients.
4. Refrigerate for up to 3 days.
5. Drizzle dressing over the salad when ready to serve.

Nutritional Content:

- Calories: 338
- Fat: 23.5
- Cholesterol: 3.8 mg
- Sodium: 57 mg
- Carbohydrates: 30.4 g
- Fiber: 3.6 g
- Sugar: 23.2 g
- Protein: 4.9 g

Broccoli Salad

Preparation Time: 15 minutes
Cooking Time: 0 minute
Servings: 4

Ingredients:

- 4 cups broccoli florets
- ½ cup almonds, sliced
- 1 cup raisins
- ½ onion, minced
- 1 cup mayonnaise
- 2 tablespoons white wine vinegar
- Pinch garlic salt

Method:

1. Mix all ingredients in food container.
2. Seal and refrigerate for up to 3 days.

Nutritional Content:

- Calories: 373.8
- Fat: 7 g
- Cholesterol: 13 mg
- Sodium: 35 mg
- Carbohydrates: 28 g
- Fiber: 3.2 g
- Sugar: 3 g
- Protein: 7.3 g

Kale Salad

Preparation Time: 15 minutes
Cooking Time: 0 minute
Servings: 4

Ingredients:

- 6 cups kale leaves
- 1 cup croutons

Dressing

- ½ cup olive oil
- ½ cup lemon juice
- ½ teaspoon Dijon mustard
- 2 cloves garlic, minced

Method:

1. Place kale leaves in food containers.
2. Top with croutons.
3. Seal and refrigerate for up to 2 days.
4. Mix dressing ingredients and add to a sauce cup.
5. Refrigerate.
6. Drizzle salad with dressing before serving.

Nutritional Content:

- Calories: 361
- Fat: 13
- Cholesterol: 6 mg
- Sodium: 437 mg
- Carbohydrates: 17.6 g
- Fiber: 2.2 g
- Sugar: 1.2 g
- Protein: 6.8 g

Mediterranean Salad

Preparation Time: 10 minutes
Cooking Time: 0 minute
Servings: 4

Ingredients:

- 2 cucumbers, sliced
- ¼ cup sun-dried tomatoes, sliced
- 2 cups tomatoes, diced
- 1 red onion, sliced
- 1 cup black olives, sliced
- 1 ½ cup feta cheese, crumbled

Method:

1. Combine all ingredients in food containers.
2. Seal and refrigerate for up to 1 day.

Nutritional Content:

- Calories: 130
- Fat: 8.8
- Cholesterol: 25 mg
- Sodium: 86 mg
- Carbohydrates: 9.3 g
- Fiber: 2.1 g
- Sugar: 4.5 g
- Protein: 5.5 g
- Cholesterol: 0 mg
- Sodium: 62 mg
- Carbohydrates: 32 g
- Fiber: 6.2 g
- Sugar: 3 g
- Protein: 6 g

Chapter 10: Drinks

Spinach & Banana Smoothie

Preparation Time: 5 minutes
Cooking Time: 0 minute
Servings: 1

Ingredients:

- 1 banana, sliced
- 1 cup spinach leaves
- 1 cup unsweetened soymilk

Method:

1. Process all ingredients in a blender.
2. Chill in the refrigerator for up to 1 day.

Nutritional Content:

- Calories: 257.4
- Fat: 4.8
- Cholesterol: 0 mg
- Sodium: 14 mg
- Carbohydrates: 47.1 g
- Fiber: 5.5 g
- Sugar: 6 g
- Protein: 10.1 g

Blackberry Lemonade

Preparation Time: 5 minutes
Cooking Time: 0 minute
Servings: 4

Ingredients:

- 1 cup blackberries
- ¾ cup Splenda
- 4 ½ cups water
- 1 cup lemon juice
- 4 cups ice cubes

Method:

1. Blend blackberries in a food processor.
2. Add pureed blackberries and the rest of the ingredients to a pitcher.
3. Refrigerate for up to 2 days.

Nutritional Content:

- Calories: 200
- Fat: 0.2 g
- Cholesterol: 0 mg
- Sodium: 15 mg
- Carbohydrates: 52.5 g
- Fiber: 2 g
- Sugar: 4 g
- Protein: 0.7 g

Green Smoothie

Preparation Time: 5 minutes
Cooking Time: 0 minute
Servings: 2

Ingredients:

- 6 leaves kale
- 2 green apples, sliced
- 1 cucumber, sliced
- 4 stalks celery
- 1 tablespoon ginger, minced
- 1 tablespoon lemon juice

Method:

1. Add all ingredients to a blender.
2. Blend until smooth.
3. Refrigerate for up to 1 day.

Nutritional Content:

- Calories: 143.5
- Fat: 1.1 g
- Cholesterol: 0 mg
- Sodium: 81 mg
- Carbohydrates: 36 g
- Fiber: 7.7 g
- Sugar: 12 g
- Protein: 4.2 g

Blueberry Smoothie

Preparation Time: 5 minutes
Cooking Time: 0 minute
Servings: 2

Ingredients:

- 1 cup blueberries
- 8 oz. yogurt
- ¾ cup nonfat milk
- 2 tablespoons Splenda
- ½ teaspoon vanilla extract
- ⅛ teaspoon ground nutmeg

Method:

1. Combine all ingredients in a blender.
2. Pulse until smooth.
3. Transfer to a pitcher
4. Refrigerate for up to 1 day.

Nutritional Content:

- Calories: 211
- Fat: 9.5 g
- Cholesterol: 0 mg
- Sodium: 17 mg
- Carbohydrates: 24 g
- Fiber: 1.8 g
- Sugar: 3 g
- Protein: 9.5 g

Watermelon Water

Preparation Time: 20 minutes
Cooking Time: 0 minute
Servings: 4

Ingredients:

- 4 cups watermelon, sliced into cubes
- 8 cups water
- 4 lime slices
- 1/8 cup mint leaves

Method:

1. Blend watermelon in a food processor.
2. Add to a pitcher with water along with lime slices and mint leaves.
3. Refrigerate for up to 3 days.

Nutritional Content:

- Calories: 25
- Fat: 0.1 g
- Cholesterol: 0 mg
- Sodium: 1.3 mg
- Carbohydrates: 18 g
- Fiber: 0.4 g
- Sugar: 17 g
- Protein: 0.5 g

Conclusion

If you have been worrying about your obesity, your figure and health, and you want to start the journey of losing weight, you want to eat low-fat but delicious food, but you don't know what kind of three meals a day to make, then this Bariatric Meal Prep cookbook is absolutely suitable for you. Follow this cookbook with straightforward instructions, encouraging advice, and time saving tips make meal planning, prep, and cooking for low-fat diet that much easier.

Thank you for buying this book. Now let's start your gourmet journey! Nourish and protect your gut with these diverse and delightful dishes!

CPSIA information can be obtained
at www.ICGtesting.com
Printed in the USA
BVHW012239270322
632576BV00003B/126